This Journal belongs to:

_____

There is a saying – you can't manage what you don't measure.

Measuring your intake helps you manage your output.

A healthier inside makes for a more attractive outside.

Become your own Boss today, by managing what you eat, and how you use those calories

Tips for using a habit tracker

- **Why**

  - Here a five compelling reasons.
  - 1. It creates a visual cue that can remind you to act.
  - 2. It is motivating to see the progress you are making.
  - 3. It motivates you to continue.
  - 4. It provides immediate satisfaction.
  - 5. Finally, tracking feels rewarding
- Tracking specific habits also helps keep you focused on the process rather
- than the result.

- **What**
  -
- **Common habits to track:**
- meditate
- write 1 thing I'm grateful for
- Exercise
- Walk the dog

- **When**
- Anytime you remember really but it has been found for some that)
  - ·

Habit Tracker

Month _____
Year

Day	Write in Journal	Meditate	Exercise										
1	▓		▓										
2		▓											
3	▓	▓	▓										
4		▓											
5	▓		▓										
6		▓	▓										
7	▓												
8													
9													
10													
11													
12													
13													
14													
15													
16													
17													
18													
19													
20													
21													
22													
23													
24													
25													
26													
27													
28													
29													
30													
31													

abit
racker

Month _____
Year _____

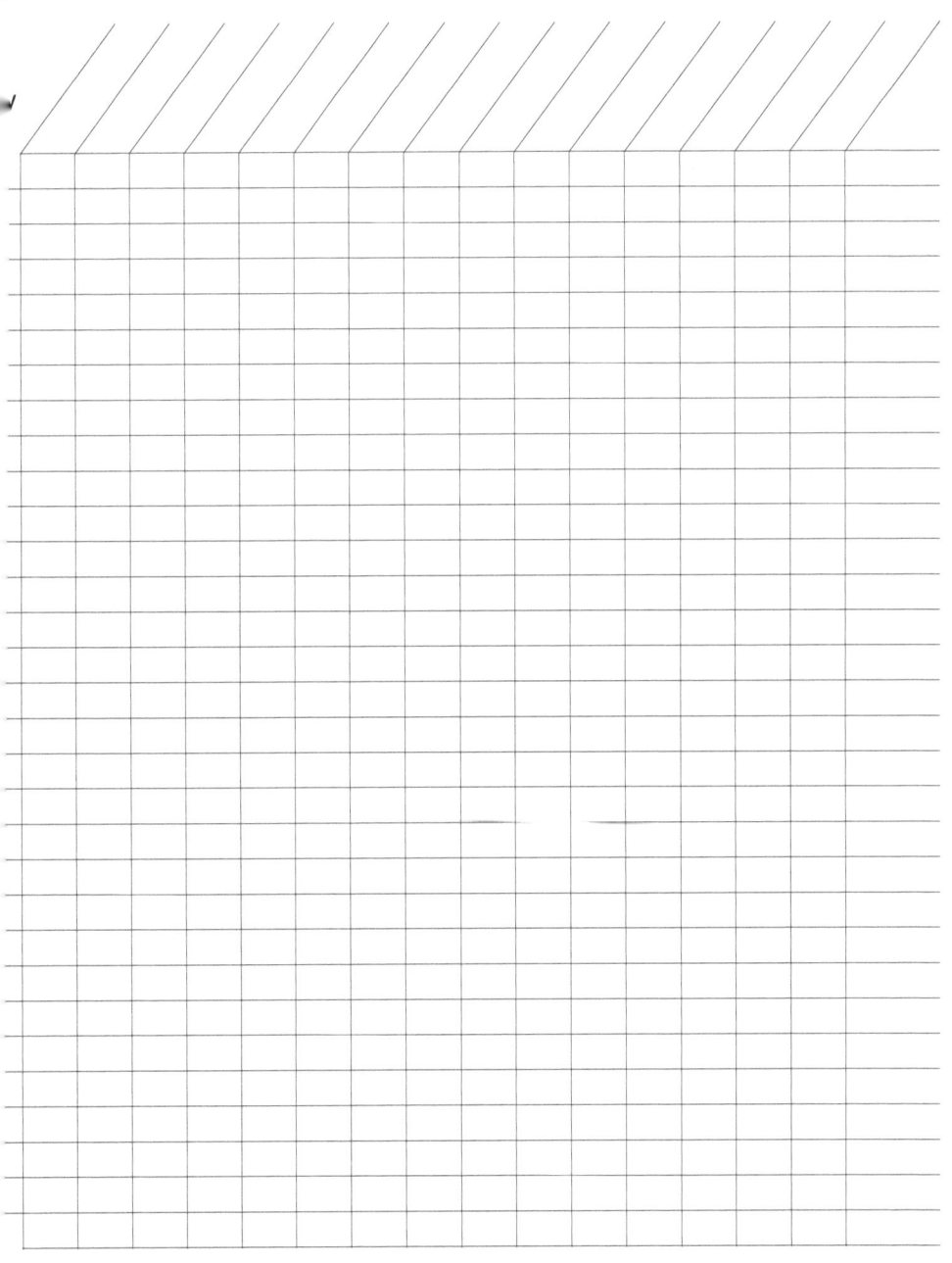

Notes:

Date	S M T W T F S	
Breakfast	Amount	Calories (kcal)
	Total	
Snack	Amount	Calories (kcal)
	Total	
Lunch	Amount	Calories (kcal)
	Total	

Snack	Amount	Calories (kcal)
	Total	
Dinner	Amount	Calories (kcal)
	Total	
Snack	Amount	Calories (kcal)
	Total	
Exercise	Duration	Calories burned (kcal)
Water	Fruit & Veggies	

Notes:

Date	S M T W T F S	
Breakfast	Amount	Calories (kcal)
	Total	
Snack	Amount	Calories (kcal)
	Total	
Lunch	Amount	Calories (kcal)
	Total	

Snack	Amount	Calories (kcal)
	Total	
Dinner	Amount	Calories (kcal)
	Total	
Snack	Amount	Calories (kcal)
	Total	
Exercise	Duration	Calories burned (kcal)

Water								Fruit & Veggies							

Notes:

Date	S M T W T F S	
Breakfast	Amount	Calories (kcal)
	Total	
Snack	Amount	Calories (kcal)
	Total	
Lunch	Amount	Calories (kcal)
	Total	

Snack	Amount	Calories (kcal)
	Total	
Dinner	Amount	Calories (kcal)
	Total	
Snack	Amount	Calories (kcal)
	Total	
Exercise	Duration	Calories burned (kcal)

Water								Fruit & Veggies							

Notes:

Date	S M T W T F S	
Breakfast	Amount	Calories (kcal)
	Total	
Snack	Amount	Calories (kcal)
	Total	
Lunch	Amount	Calories (kcal)
	Total	

Snack	Amount	Calories (kcal)
	Total	
Dinner	Amount	Calories (kcal)
	Total	
Snack	Amount	Calories (kcal)
	Total	
Exercise	Duration	Calories burned (kcal)

Water								Fruit & Veggies								

Notes:

Date	S M T W T F S	
Breakfast	Amount	Calories (kcal)
	Total	
Snack	Amount	Calories (kcal)
	Total	
Lunch	Amount	Calories (kcal)
	Total	

Snack	Amount	Calories (kcal)
	Total	
Dinner	Amount	Calories (kcal)
	Total	
Snack	Amount	Calories (kcal)
	Total	
Exercise	Duration	Calories burned (kcal)

Water								Fruit & Veggies						

Notes:

Date		S M T W T F S	
Breakfast		Amount	Calories (kcal)
		Total	
Snack		Amount	Calories (kcal)
		Total	
Lunch		Amount	Calories (kcal)
		Total	

Snack	Amount	Calories (kcal)
	Total	
Dinner	Amount	Calories (kcal)
	Total	
Snack	Amount	Calories (kcal)
	Total	
Exercise	Duration	Calories burned (kcal)
Water		Fruit & Veggies

Notes:

Date	S M T W T F S	
Breakfast	Amount	Calories (kcal)
	Total	
Snack	Amount	Calories (kcal)
	Total	
Lunch	Amount	Calories (kcal)
	Total	

Snack	Amount	Calories (kcal)
	Total	
Dinner	Amount	Calories (kcal)
	Total	
Snack	Amount	Calories (kcal)
	Total	
Exercise	Duration	Calories burned (kcal)
Water									Fruit & Veggies								

Notes:

Date	S M T W T F S	
Breakfast	Amount	Calories (kcal)
	Total	
Snack	Amount	Calories (kcal)
	Total	
Lunch	Amount	Calories (kcal)
	Total	

Snack	Amount	Calories (kcal)
	Total	
Dinner	Amount	Calories (kcal)
	Total	
Snack	Amount	Calories (kcal)
	Total	
Exercise	Duration	Calories burned (kcal)

Water									Fruit & Veggies								

Notes:

Date	S M T W T F S	
Breakfast	Amount	Calories (kcal)
	Total	
Snack	Amount	Calories (kcal)
	Total	
Lunch	Amount	Calories (kcal)
	Total	

Snack	Amount	Calories (kcal)
	Total	

Dinner	Amount	Calories (kcal)
	Total	

Snack	Amount	Calories (kcal)
	Total	

Exercise	Duration	Calories burned (kcal)

Water								Fruit & Veggies							

Notes:

Date	S M T W T F S	
Breakfast	Amount	Calories (kcal)
	Total	
Snack	Amount	Calories (kcal)
	Total	
Lunch	Amount	Calories (kcal)
	Total	

Snack	Amount	Calories (kcal)
	Total	
Dinner	Amount	Calories (kcal)
	Total	
Snack	Amount	Calories (kcal)
	Total	
Exercise	Duration	Calories burned (kcal)
Water		Fruit & Veggies	

Notes:

Date	S M T W T F S	
Breakfast	Amount	Calories (kcal)
	Total	
Snack	Amount	Calories (kcal)
	Total	
Lunch	Amount	Calories (kcal)
	Total	

Snack	Amount	Calories (kcal)
	Total	
Dinner	Amount	Calories (kcal)
	Total	
Snack	Amount	Calories (kcal)
	Total	
Exercise	Duration	Calories burned (kcal)
Water										Fruit & Veggies									

Notes:

Date		S M T W T F S	
Breakfast	Amount	Calories (kcal)	
	Total		
Snack	Amount	Calories (kcal)	
	Total		
Lunch	Amount	Calories (kcal)	
	Total		

Snack	Amount	Calories (kcal)
	Total	
Dinner	Amount	Calories (kcal)
	Total	
Snack	Amount	Calories (kcal)
	Total	
Exercise	Duration	Calories burned (kcal)

Water								Fruit & Veggies							

Notes:

Date	S M T W T F S	
Breakfast	Amount	Calories (kcal)
	Total	
Snack	Amount	Calories (kcal)
	Total	
Lunch	Amount	Calories (kcal)
	Total	

Snack	Amount	Calories (kcal)
	Total	
Dinner	Amount	Calories (kcal)
	Total	
Snack	Amount	Calories (kcal)
	Total	
Exercise	Duration	Calories burned (kcal)
Water	Fruit & Veggies	

Notes:

Date	S M T W T F S	
Breakfast	Amount	Calories (kcal)
	Total	
Snack	Amount	Calories (kcal)
	Total	
Lunch	Amount	Calories (kcal)
	Total	

Snack	Amount	Calories (kcal)
	Total	
Dinner	Amount	Calories (kcal)
	Total	
Snack	Amount	Calories (kcal)
	Total	
Exercise	Duration	Calories burned (kcal)
Water		Fruit & Veggies

Notes:

Date	S M T W T F S	
Breakfast	Amount	Calories (kcal)
	Total	
Snack	Amount	Calories (kcal)
	Total	
Lunch	Amount	Calories (kcal)
	Total	

Snack	Amount	Calories (kcal)
	Total	
Dinner	Amount	Calories (kcal)
	Total	
Snack	Amount	Calories (kcal)
	Total	
Exercise	Duration	Calories burned (kcal)
Water								Fruit & Veggies							

Notes:

Date		S M T W T F S	
Breakfast	Amount	Calories (kcal)	
	Total		
Snack	Amount	Calories (kcal)	
	Total		
Lunch	Amount	Calories (kcal)	
	Total		

Snack	Amount	Calories (kcal)
	Total	
Dinner	Amount	Calories (kcal)
	Total	
Snack	Amount	Calories (kcal)
	Total	
Exercise	Duration	Calories burned (kcal)

Water									Fruit & Veggies								

Notes:

Date		S M T W T F S	
Breakfast	Amount	Calories (kcal)	
	Total		
Snack	Amount	Calories (kcal)	
	Total		
Lunch	Amount	Calories (kcal)	
	Total		

Snack	Amount	Calories (kcal)
	Total	
Dinner	Amount	Calories (kcal)
	Total	
Snack	Amount	Calories (kcal)
	Total	
Exercise	Duration	Calories burned (kcal)
Water	Fruit & Veggies	

Notes:

Date	S M T W T F S	
Breakfast	Amount	Calories (kcal)
	Total	
Snack	Amount	Calories (kcal)
	Total	
Lunch	Amount	Calories (kcal)
	Total	

Snack	Amount	Calories (kcal)
	Total	
Dinner	Amount	Calories (kcal)
	Total	
Snack	Amount	Calories (kcal)
	Total	
Exercise	Duration	Calories burned (kcal)

Water							Fruit & Veggies							

Notes:

Date		S M T W T F S
Breakfast	Amount	Calories (kcal)
	Total	
Snack	Amount	Calories (kcal)
	Total	
Lunch	Amount	Calories (kcal)
	Total	

Snack	Amount	Calories (kcal)
	Total	
Dinner	Amount	Calories (kcal)
	Total	
Snack	Amount	Calories (kcal)
	Total	
Exercise	Duration	Calories burned (kcal)
Water									Fruit & Veggies								

Notes:

Date		S M T W T F S	
Breakfast		Amount	Calories (kcal)
		Total	
Snack		Amount	Calories (kcal)
		Total	
Lunch		Amount	Calories (kcal)
		Total	

Snack	Amount	Calories (kcal)
	Total	
Dinner	Amount	Calories (kcal)
	Total	
Snack	Amount	Calories (kcal)
	Total	
Exercise	Duration	Calories burned (kcal)

Water		Fruit & Veggies	

Notes:

Date		S M T W T F S	
Breakfast	Amount		Calories (kcal)
	Total		
Snack	Amount		Calories (kcal)
	Total		
Lunch	Amount		Calories (kcal)
	Total		

Snack	Amount	Calories (kcal)
	Total	
Dinner	Amount	Calories (kcal)
	Total	
Snack	Amount	Calories (kcal)
	Total	
Exercise	Duration	Calories burned (kcal)

Water								Fruit & Veggies							

Notes:

Date		S M T W T F S	
Breakfast		Amount	Calories (kcal)
		Total	
Snack		Amount	Calories (kcal)
		Total	
Lunch		Amount	Calories (kcal)
		Total	

Snack	Amount	Calories (kcal)
	Total	
Dinner	Amount	Calories (kcal)
	Total	
Snack	Amount	Calories (kcal)
	Total	
Exercise	Duration	Calories burned (kcal)
Water		Fruit & Veggies	

Notes:

Date		S M T W T F S
Breakfast	Amount	Calories (kcal)
	Total	
Snack	Amount	Calories (kcal)
	Total	
Lunch	Amount	Calories (kcal)
	Total	

Snack	Amount	Calories (kcal)
	Total	
Dinner	Amount	Calories (kcal)
	Total	
Snack	Amount	Calories (kcal)
	Total	
Exercise	Duration	Calories burned (kcal)
Water	Fruit & Veggies	

Notes:

Date	S M T W T F S	
Breakfast	Amount	Calories (kcal)
	Total	
Snack	Amount	Calories (kcal)
	Total	
Lunch	Amount	Calories (kcal)
	Total	

Snack	Amount	Calories (kcal)
	Total	
Dinner	Amount	Calories (kcal)
	Total	
Snack	Amount	Calories (kcal)
	Total	
Exercise	Duration	Calories burned (kcal)

Water								Fruit & Veggies								

Notes:

Date	S M T W T F S	
Breakfast	Amount	Calories (kcal)
	Total	
Snack	Amount	Calories (kcal)
	Total	
Lunch	Amount	Calories (kcal)
	Total	

Snack	Amount	Calories (kcal)
	Total	
Dinner	Amount	Calories (kcal)
	Total	
Snack	Amount	Calories (kcal)
	Total	
Exercise	Duration	Calories burned (kcal)
Water	Fruit & Veggies	

Notes:

Date		S M T W T F S	
Breakfast	Amount		Calories (kcal)
	Total		
Snack	Amount		Calories (kcal)
	Total		
Lunch	Amount		Calories (kcal)
	Total		

Snack	Amount	Calories (kcal)
	Total	
Dinner	Amount	Calories (kcal)
	Total	
Snack	Amount	Calories (kcal)
	Total	
Exercise	Duration	Calories burned (kcal)
Water		Fruit & Veggies		

Notes:

Date		S M T W T F S
Breakfast	Amount	Calories (kcal)
	Total	
Snack	Amount	Calories (kcal)
	Total	
Lunch	Amount	Calories (kcal)
	Total	

Snack	Amount	Calories (kcal)
	Total	
Dinner	Amount	Calories (kcal)
	Total	
Snack	Amount	Calories (kcal)
	Total	
Exercise	Duration	Calories burned (kcal)
Water	Fruit & Veggies	

Notes:

Date	S M T W T F S	
Breakfast	Amount	Calories (kcal)
	Total	
Snack	Amount	Calories (kcal)
	Total	
Lunch	Amount	Calories (kcal)
	Total	

Snack	Amount	Calories (kcal)
	Total	
Dinner	Amount	Calories (kcal)
	Total	
Snack	Amount	Calories (kcal)
	Total	
Exercise	Duration	Calories burned (kcal)
Water		Fruit & Veggies

Notes:

Date		S M T W T F S	
Breakfast		Amount	Calories (kcal)
		Total	
Snack		Amount	Calories (kcal)
		Total	
Lunch		Amount	Calories (kcal)
		Total	

Snack	Amount	Calories (kcal)
	Total	
Dinner	Amount	Calories (kcal)
	Total	
Snack	Amount	Calories (kcal)
	Total	
Exercise	Duration	Calories burned (kcal)

Water								Fruit & Veggies							

Notes:

Date		S M T W T F S	
Breakfast	Amount		Calories (kcal)
	Total		
Snack	Amount		Calories (kcal)
	Total		
Lunch	Amount		Calories (kcal)
	Total		

Snack	Amount	Calories (kcal)
	Total	
Dinner	Amount	Calories (kcal)
	Total	
Snack	Amount	Calories (kcal)
	Total	
Exercise	Duration	Calories burned (kcal)

| Water | | | | | | | | Fruit & Veggies | | | | | | | | |

Notes:

Date	S M T W T F S	
Breakfast	Amount	Calories (kcal)
	Total	
Snack	Amount	Calories (kcal)
	Total	
Lunch	Amount	Calories (kcal)
	Total	

Snack	Amount	Calories (kcal)
	Total	

Dinner	Amount	Calories (kcal)
	Total	

Snack	Amount	Calories (kcal)
	Total	

Exercise	Duration	Calories burned (kcal)

Water								Fruit & Veggies							

Notes:

Date		S M T W T F S	
Breakfast	Amount		Calories (kcal)
	Total		
Snack	Amount		Calories (kcal)
	Total		
Lunch	Amount		Calories (kcal)
	Total		

Snack	Amount	Calories (kcal)
	Total	
Dinner	Amount	Calories (kcal)
	Total	
Snack	Amount	Calories (kcal)
	Total	
Exercise	Duration	Calories burned (kcal)

Water									Fruit & Veggies							

Notes:

Date	S M T W T F S	
Breakfast	Amount	Calories (kcal)
	Total	
Snack	Amount	Calories (kcal)
	Total	
Lunch	Amount	Calories (kcal)
	Total	

Snack	Amount	Calories (kcal)
	Total	
Dinner	Amount	Calories (kcal)
	Total	
Snack	Amount	Calories (kcal)
	Total	
Exercise	Duration	Calories burned (kcal)
Water								Fruit & Veggies							

Notes:

Date	S M T W T F S	
Breakfast	Amount	Calories (kcal)
	Total	
Snack	Amount	Calories (kcal)
	Total	
Lunch	Amount	Calories (kcal)
	Total	

Snack	Amount	Calories (kcal)
	Total	
Dinner	Amount	Calories (kcal)
	Total	
Snack	Amount	Calories (kcal)
	Total	
Exercise	Duration	Calories burned (kcal)
Water		Fruit & Veggies	

Notes:

Date	S M T W T F S	
Breakfast	Amount	Calories (kcal)
	Total	
Snack	Amount	Calories (kcal)
	Total	
Lunch	Amount	Calories (kcal)
	Total	

Snack	Amount	Calories (kcal)
	Total	
Dinner	Amount	Calories (kcal)
	Total	
Snack	Amount	Calories (kcal)
	Total	
Exercise	Duration	Calories burned (kcal)
Water	Fruit & Veggies	

Notes:

Date		S M T W T F S	
Breakfast	Amount	Calories (kcal)	
	Total		
Snack	Amount	Calories (kcal)	
	Total		
Lunch	Amount	Calories (kcal)	
	Total		

Snack	Amount	Calories (kcal)
	Total	
Dinner	Amount	Calories (kcal)
	Total	
Snack	Amount	Calories (kcal)
	Total	
Exercise	Duration	Calories burned (kcal)

| Water | | | | | | | | | Fruit & Veggies | | | | | | | | |

Notes:

Date		S M T W T F S	
Breakfast		Amount	Calories (kcal)
		Total	
Snack		Amount	Calories (kcal)
		Total	
Lunch		Amount	Calories (kcal)
		Total	

Snack	Amount	Calories (kcal)
	Total	
Dinner	Amount	Calories (kcal)
	Total	
Snack	Amount	Calories (kcal)
	Total	
Exercise	Duration	Calories burned (kcal)
Water	Fruit & Veggies	

Notes:

Date	S M T W T F S	
Breakfast	Amount	Calories (kcal)
	Total	
Snack	Amount	Calories (kcal)
	Total	
Lunch	Amount	Calories (kcal)
	Total	

Snack	Amount	Calories (kcal)
	Total	
Dinner	Amount	Calories (kcal)
	Total	
Snack	Amount	Calories (kcal)
	Total	
Exercise	Duration	Calories burned (kcal)

Water								Fruit & Veggies							

Notes:

Date	S M T W T F S	
Breakfast	Amount	Calories (kcal)
	Total	
Snack	Amount	Calories (kcal)
	Total	
Lunch	Amount	Calories (kcal)
	Total	

Snack	Amount	Calories (kcal)
	Total	
Dinner	Amount	Calories (kcal)
	Total	
Snack	Amount	Calories (kcal)
	Total	
Exercise	Duration	Calories burned (kcal)
Water									Fruit & Veggies							

Notes:

Date	S M T W T F S	
Breakfast	Amount	Calories (kcal)
	Total	
Snack	Amount	Calories (kcal)
	Total	
Lunch	Amount	Calories (kcal)
	Total	

Snack	Amount	Calories (kcal)
	Total	
Dinner	Amount	Calories (kcal)
	Total	
Snack	Amount	Calories (kcal)
	Total	
Exercise	Duration	Calories burned (kcal)
Water		Fruit & Veggies

www.ingramcontent.com/pod-product-compliance
Lightning Source LLC
Chambersburg PA
CBHW051352280526
45784CB00007B/2921